I0782856

INTEGRAL AROMATHERAPY

Science, emotion and spirit

in the art of essential oils

ELIAS H. VARENZA

CONTENT

INTRODUCTION

<u>Welcome to the World of Integral Aromatherapy</u>

Welcome to the fascinating world of integral aromatherapy, a practice that invites us to rediscover the power of aromas to balance the body, mind and spirit. Since ancient times, natural essences have accompanied human beings in their rituals of healing, well-being and spiritual connection.

Today, thanks to advances in science and the growing search for holistic wellness methods, aromatherapy has become an art and a science, capable of transforming our environment and our emotions in profound ways.

This book is born with the desire to offer you a complete guide, where the scientific foundations of aromatherapy, its emotional impact and its potential in spiritual life converge. Here you will discover how each aroma hides a door to a particular state of well-being, capable of relaxing you, energizing you or helping you find mental clarity in moments of uncertainty.

I invite you to explore this aromatic universe from a comprehensive and conscious perspective, connecting with the power of essences in a unique and meaningful way.

Objectives of the Book: Science, Emotion and Spirituality in the Use of Essential Oils

This book has three main objectives: to teach you the scientific foundations that support aromatherapy, to guide you in the emotional use of essential oils and to accompany you in spiritual exploration through aromas.

*** Science:** Throughout these pages, we will delve into the biochemical components of essential oils and their effect on the nervous system and emotions. You will understand how the sense of smell, in connection with the limbic system, can influence your mood, reduce stress and improve health in tangible ways.

*** Emotion:** Aromatherapy is also a powerful tool for managing emotions. You will learn how certain essential oils can bring you calm in times of anxiety, relief in times of sadness, or energy in times of emotional exhaustion. Here you will find practical blends and techniques to improve your emotional well-being.

*** Spirituality:** In addition to its scientific and emotional effect, aromatherapy offers us a door to the spiritual world. You will explore how aromas can be used in meditation, energy balance, and introspection. This book will help you connect with your inner self through rituals and practices that integrate essential oils into your spiritual life.

By combining these three approaches, this book will allow you to understand the art of aromatherapy in all its dimensions, offering you a complete path to comprehensive well-being.

How to Benefit from this Guide: Practices, Principles and Applications

To get the most out of this book, I encourage you to approach each section in a practical and thoughtful way. This is not just a reference manual, but an invitation to experiment, explore, and make aromatherapy a personal and unique tool. Here are some tips for navigating this guide:

Dive into the scientific principles: The first few chapters are designed to help you understand the basics of essential oils and their impact on the body and mind. Feel free to read and reread these concepts; the better you understand them, the more you will benefit from each practical application.

Try suggested practices and blends: As you progress, you will find recipes and techniques for using essential oils in specific ways. Take the time to try each blend and see how your body and mood respond to each scent. Aromatherapy is, above all, a personal experience that requires attention and sensitivity.

Integrate aromatherapy into your routine: This book offers you tools to include essential oils in your daily life, whether at home, at work or in moments of introspection. Make this practice an ally in your daily life and see how you can progressively transform your environment and your emotions.

I hope this book will become a reliable companion and a source of inspiration on your journey to holistic wellness. May the scents awaken in you a deeper connection with yourself and the world around you.

PART I

FUNDAMENTALS OF SCIENTIFIC AROMATHERAPY

CHAPTER 1

ESSENTIAL OILS AND THEIR ORIGINS

This chapter delves into the fascinating process by which plants offer us their purest essences, transforming them into essential oils. Knowing the process from plant to bottle is essential to understanding their therapeutic value, as each extraction step, each choice of plant and each purification process defines the quality and potential of the essential oil. We will explore how essential oils capture the essence of nature, keeping their properties intact so that we can experience their power in every application.

<u>Extraction and Purity of Essential Oils</u>

The process of extracting essential oils is as important as the choice of the plant itself, as it determines the quality, purity and chemical profile of the oil. The effectiveness of aromatherapy depends on the precision with which this extraction is carried out. Let's look in detail at each method and its implications:

Steam Distillation:

Process and Applications: Steam distillation is one of the oldest methods and is still the most widely used. This process begins with the introduction of steam into a chamber containing the plant. The steam penetrates the cell walls of the plant, releasing the aromatic molecules which are mixed with the steam and then cooled in a condenser.

Finally, they are separated into two phases: water and oil. Distillation is ideal for aromatic plants such as rosemary, eucalyptus and thyme.

Impact on Purity: Distillation at appropriate temperatures allows the sensitive components of the plant to be maintained, preserving its chemical composition. A good distiller knows how to manage times and temperatures, since any variation can affect the quality of the oil.

Example in Practice: A lavender essential oil obtained through steam distillation offers a chemical profile that retains its calming properties. This method is ideal for oils that are applied topically or inhaled for relaxing effects.

Cold Pressed:

Process and Applications: Used primarily for citrus fruits, cold pressing involves pressing the peel of the fruit to release the essential oils without the need for heat. This method preserves the fresh and vibrant aromas characteristic of citrus fruits, making them ideal for use in diffusers and energizing formulations.

Unique Benefits: By not subjecting it to heat, cold pressing keeps the volatile compounds in their natural state, resulting in a much purer and fresher aroma.

Example in Practice: A cold-pressed lemon essential oil is commonly used in blends to increase concentration and reduce fatigue.

Supercritical CO_2 Extraction:

Process and Applications: This method uses supercritical carbon dioxide, a physical state between liquid and gas, to extract aromatic compounds. It is a sophisticated process that requires specialized equipment, but results in an oil of extremely high purity, without solvent residues.

User Benefits: Oils extracted with CO_2 **retain** a broader spectrum of aromatic molecules, enhancing their therapeutic and aromatic benefits. In addition, this method is safe for the environment, as it leaves no toxic residues.

Example in Practice: CO_2 extracted frankincense essential oil is particularly useful in meditation and introspection due to its ability to help calm the mind.

<u>Sustainable and Ethical Practices in Oil Extraction</u>

The production of essential oils has a significant impact on the environment. Adopting sustainable practices not only protects the quality of the oils, but also contributes to preserving natural resources for future generations.

Below we discuss practices and certifications that ensure environmentally friendly production:

Sustainable Harvesting and Plant Selection:

Importance: Sustainable harvesting involves harvesting plants at their optimal point of ripeness and at specific periods that allow for natural regeneration. Careful selection of plants ensures that the oils maintain their therapeutic potency without overexploiting natural resources.

Practice Example: In some communities, sandalwood harvesting is done respecting growth cycles and avoiding cutting down young trees, ensuring that the ecosystem remains balanced.

Transparency and Traceability in Production:

Definition : Traceability allows each bottle of essential oil to be tracked from its origin to the final consumer, offering security over the entire process.

User Benefit: Transparency helps users make informed decisions about the oils they purchase, confident that they are getting a quality product that respects both the environment and the people involved in its production.

Ethical and Ecological Certifications:

Key Certificates: Certifications such as "Organic" and "Fair Trade" ensure that oils come from crops without pesticides and with trade practices that benefit workers.

Example in Practice: A certified organic peppermint essential oil is ideal for those looking for a chemical-free alternative that supports ethical farming practices.

The Chemistry of Oils: What Makes Them Unique?

The chemistry of essential oils is one of the reasons for their effectiveness. Each oil contains a blend of unique compounds that interact synergistically, producing therapeutic effects. Let's look at the main chemical families and their therapeutic properties:

Monoterpenes:

Examples and Properties: Present in oils such as lemon and pine, monoterpenes have anti-inflammatory and immune-boosting properties. They are useful in purification and revitalizing blends.

Practical Application: Oils rich in monoterpenes are ideal for people looking to improve their physical endurance and vitality.

Esters:

Examples and Properties: Lavender and bergamot contain esters, compounds known for their relaxing and antispasmodic capacity.

Practical Application: Ester-rich oils are frequently used in formulas to relieve anxiety and insomnia, as they induce a feeling of calm.

Phenols:

Examples and Properties: Phenols, such as carvacrol in oregano, are highly antimicrobial, offering effective protection against bacteria and fungi.

Practical Application: They are effective in formulations for the immune system and for disinfection, although they require adequate dilutions due to their potency.

Terpene Alcohols :

Examples and Properties : Linalool in lavender has balancing and antiseptic properties, making it ideal for skin care and emotional balance.

Practical Application : Their gentleness makes them an excellent choice for topical treatments on sensitive skin.

CHAPTER 2

THE OLFACTORY SYSTEM AND ITS EFFECTS ON THE BRAIN

The olfactory system is a fascinating and unique pathway through which essential oils interact directly with our brain and, consequently, with our emotions, memory and moods. Unlike the other senses, smell has a direct connection with the limbic system, which is responsible for our emotional responses and memories. This chapter explores how aromas are processed in the brain, how they influence our emotions and how aromatherapy becomes an effective tool for managing emotional and mental well-being.

<u>How the Sense of Smell Connects with Our Emotions</u>

The sense of smell has the unique ability to trigger immediate emotional reactions. When we inhale a scent, the aromatic molecules enter through the nose and reach the olfactory receptors, where they interact with specialized cells that send signals to different areas of the brain, especially the limbic system, the region responsible for emotion, motivation and memory.

The Direct Olfactory Route to the Brain:

Unlike other senses, such as sight or touch, which must pass through several areas of the brain before reaching the limbic system, smell has a direct connection to this region. This proximity explains why scents generate such immediate and powerful emotional responses. Within seconds, the aroma we inhale can trigger memories, change our mood, and evoke intense emotions.

This direct route also allows aromas to influence the nervous system quickly, modulating brain activity and affecting neurotransmitters such as serotonin and GABA, which play a fundamental role in regulating anxiety and emotional well-being.

Examples of Emotional Connections with Aromas:

Studies show that the scent of lavender is able to reduce anxiety and promote calm by activating olfactory receptors that influence the amygdala, a key region in the processing of emotions. On the other hand, the scent of mint has an energizing effect and can stimulate the central nervous system, increasing alertness and concentration.

Another example is the scent of the rose, which has a long history of being used in meditative practices and emotional healing rituals. This scent, when inhaled, sends signals that reduce the production of cortisol, the stress hormone, inducing a state of relaxation.

The Science Behind the Brain's Response to Scents

Each scent has the ability to affect brain chemistry. The active compounds in essential oils interact with the brain in different ways, generating specific effects that can be harnessed to treat certain emotional and psychological imbalances. Here we explore how certain oils can influence neurotransmitters and how this translates into a specific emotional response.

The Influence of Neurotransmitters:

Serotonin : This neurotransmitter is essential for emotional balance and mood regulation. Some oils, such as bergamot and lavender, can stimulate the release of serotonin, helping to reduce anxiety and improve feelings of well-being.

Dopamine : Linked to motivation, focus, and pleasure, dopamine can be stimulated by aromas such as mint and rosemary, which increase mental clarity and energy levels. Dopamine helps improve concentration and is helpful in times of mental fatigue.

GABA (gamma-aminobutyric acid): This neurotransmitter inhibits the overexcitation of neurons, helping to relax the nervous system. Lavender and valerian oils could increase GABA activity, which produces calming effects and helps reduce stress.

Amygdala Activation:

The amygdala is a small structure within the limbic system that plays a crucial role in processing emotions such as fear, anger, and anxiety. When we smell a scent, the amygdala interprets the signal and triggers emotional responses. This explains why certain scents can trigger immediate responses of relaxation or alertness.

Example in Practice: During a stressful situation, inhaling a calming aroma such as chamomile or incense can help reduce the amygdala's reaction, achieving a relaxing effect that decreases the body's "fight or flight" response.

The Hypothalamus and Stress Regulation:

The hypothalamus is another region of the brain that is influenced by aromas. This organ regulates vital functions such as heart rate, blood pressure, and the endocrine system. Exposure to certain essential oils can affect the hypothalamus, helping to regulate the release of hormones such as cortisol and adrenaline, which are key in the stress response.

Stress-Regulating Oils: The aroma of ylang-ylang, for example, reduces heart rate and lowers blood pressure by acting on the hypothalamus, making it an ideal oil for people looking to balance their stress levels naturally.

The Limbic System and Aromatic Memory

Aromatic memory is one of the most powerful memories we possess. This phenomenon occurs because the olfactory system is directly connected to the hippocampus, the region of the brain responsible for storing memories. This means that aromas have the ability to transport us to specific moments in our lives, awakening memories and associated emotions.

The Relationship between Smell and Memories:

Every time we experience a significant aroma, the brain stores an olfactory trace along with sensory and emotional information from the moment. When we perceive that aroma again, the hippocampus recovers the memory and recreates the sensations of the moment experienced.

Example in Practice: The scent of a particular plant can evoke childhood memories, such as lavender in a loved one's garden. This ability of scents to evoke emotional memories allows aromatherapy to be used in emotional healing therapies and in strengthening emotional bonds.

Emotional Memory and its Therapeutic Applications:

The emotional memory associated with aromas is used in therapies to help people process past experiences and improve their emotional well-being. For example, in palliative care settings or in grief counselling, aromas can evoke positive memories and create an atmosphere of calm and serenity.

Oils that Support Emotional Healing: Frankincense and myrrh are essential oils that have traditionally been used in healing rituals. In modern aromatherapy, these scents can be used to help people connect with memories of peace and serenity.

The Impact of Aromas on Mental Health and Overall Wellbeing

Aromatherapy is a powerful tool for managing emotional well-being. Thanks to their ability to influence the brain and neurotransmitter chemistry, essential oils can be applied in a complementary way to improve mood, reduce stress, and support mental well-being.

Essential Oils for Anxiety and Stress:

Lavender, frankincense, and chamomile are some of the most studied oils for anxiety relief. These oils work by reducing amygdala activity and elevating GABA levels, which produces a feeling of deep calm.

Application Example: In a diffuser, these oils can create a relaxing environment that helps reduce stress at home or in the workplace.

Oils for Motivation and Energy:

Oils such as peppermint and rosemary are known for their stimulating properties, which can improve focus and mental clarity. Their action on the nervous system helps reduce mental fatigue and improve concentration.

Application Example: In situations where high concentration is required, such as studying or work, these oils can be used to enhance mental performance.

Improved Sleep and Rest:

Lack of sleep can aggravate stress and anxiety, affecting overall well-being. Oils such as lavender, cedarwood and vetiver have sedative properties and are effective in creating an atmosphere of rest and relaxation.

Application Example: Applying a few drops of lavender to your pillow before bed can improve sleep quality by inducing a calm state in the nervous system.

PART II

THE EMOTIONAL POWER OF AROMA

CHAPTER 3

AROMA PSYCHOLOGY: HOW AROMAS IMPACT THE MIND

Aromas have the power to alter our emotional state in profound and subtle ways. Since ancient times, civilizations have used aromatic plants and essential oils not only for their physical benefits, but also for their emotional effects. In this chapter, we will explore the connection between scents and emotions, as well as the essential oils best suited for specific emotional states such as anxiety, stress and the search for emotional balance.

<u>Relationship between Aromas and Emotions</u>

The relationship between smell and emotions is due to the direct connection between the olfactory system and the limbic system, the region of the brain responsible for emotional regulation, motivation and memory. When we inhale a smell, this aromatic journey reaches the limbic system in a matter of seconds, activating different chemical reactions in the brain that translate into emotions and moods.

The Science Behind Emotional Responses to Scents:

Each scent contains unique molecules that trigger specific responses in the brain. For example, the scent of lavender activates receptors that promote relaxation, while peppermint stimulates receptors that increase energy and focus. These responses are not coincidental;

they are linked to the chemical nature of each oil and its ability to interact with specific neurotransmitters and receptors in the brain.

Practical Example: By inhaling a relaxing aroma such as incense, studies have shown a reduction in cortisol levels (the stress hormone) in the body, which helps calm the mind and reduces symptoms of anxiety.

How Aromas Can Help Change Your Mood:

Aromatherapy offers a powerful resource for modulating emotional state on a day-to-day basis. Through the intentional use of certain oils, it is possible to influence mood, energy, and emotional stability. This is because essential oils affect neurotransmitters such as serotonin and GABA, promoting calm, focus, or revitalization.

Example in Practice: If a person is feeling anxious before a presentation, they can inhale lavender and bergamot oils to calm the mind and create a sense of security. Conversely, if they need an energy boost, a drop of peppermint on their wrists can improve their alertness.

Essential Oils for Emotional States: Anxiety, Stress and Emotional Balance

Each essential oil has specific properties that help modulate different emotions. Below are some of the most effective essential oils for managing emotional states, along with their effects on well-being.

Anxiety:

Lavender: Lavender is one of the most researched essential oils in the field of anxiety. Its calming effects help reduce activity in the central nervous system, leading to a feeling of relaxation. Studies have shown that inhaling lavender decreases anxiety by activating relaxing neurotransmitters.

Frankincense: This essential oil is helpful in reducing anxiety and promoting a connection to the present moment. Frankincense is known for its ability to induce calm and generate an atmosphere of inner peace.

Example of Use: Applying a few drops of lavender and incense in a diffuser at the end of the day can create a calm and relaxing environment at home, ideal for reducing anxiety before sleeping.

Stress

Bergamot: This oil is great for reducing stress and improving mood. Bergamot contains compounds that activate the parasympathetic system, which helps the body relax and lower blood pressure.

Ylang-Ylang: With a sweet, floral aroma, ylang-ylang is known for its calming effects and ability to lower blood pressure. It is ideal for calming nerves and reducing built-up tension.

Example of Use: A blend of bergamot and ylang-ylang in a diffuser can help reduce stress throughout the day. If applied to the wrists, this combination also serves as a relaxing natural perfume.

Emotional Balance:

Rose: Rose essential oil is valuable for promoting emotional balance. Its aroma is known to boost mood, provide comfort in times of sadness, and aid self-acceptance.

Geranium: This oil is used to harmonize emotions and promote emotional stability. Geranium is a balancing oil that is associated with emotional support and reducing sadness.

Example of Use: Topical application of a few drops of rose or geranium on the chest or neck can help balance emotions, especially during times of emotional instability.

CHAPTER 4

ESSENTIAL OILS FOR MENTAL AND EMOTIONAL WELLBEING

Essential oils can influence our emotional and mental well-being in unique and powerful ways. Beyond their aroma, each essential oil provides specific properties that can calm the mind, elevate mood, enhance concentration, and promote a state of emotional balance.

In this chapter, we will explore specific essential oil blends for calming, uplifting and mental clarity. We will also delve into breathing exercises that enhance the effects of the oils and introspective questions designed to help the reader connect with their emotions.

Blends for Calm, Mood and Mental Clarity

Creating essential oil blends is an art. Blends of oil not only amplify their individual effects, but also allow you to tailor the experience to your emotional needs at any given moment.

The following are formulas that the reader can use in different circumstances to enhance their mental and emotional well-being.

Deep Calm Blend:

Ingredients: 5 drops of lavender, 3 drops of frankincense, 2 drops of Roman chamomile, 1 drop of ylang-ylang

Properties and Benefits: This combination is excellent for reducing stress and promoting deep mental calm. Lavender is known for its calming properties, while frankincense helps to relax the mind and promote introspection. Roman chamomile brings a sense of peace and serenity, and ylang-ylang balances emotions by reducing anxiety.

Practical Uses: Diffusing the blend before bed helps prepare the mind and body for rest. It can also be applied diluted to the wrists or neck during the day to reduce nervousness.

Blend to Improve Mood and Joy

Ingredients: 4 drops of sweet orange, 3 drops of bergamot, 2 drops of rose, 2 drops of geranium

Properties and Benefits: This citrus and floral blend is ideal for lifting the spirits and providing a sense of optimism. Sweet orange is energizing and cheerful, while bergamot balances emotions and reduces feelings of sadness. Rose and geranium offer emotional comfort and help open the heart, promoting a positive attitude.

Practical Uses: Ideal for those days when one needs an emotional boost. Can be used in a diffuser or diluted in a base oil to apply to the chest, promoting a feeling of well-being and relief.

Blend for Mental Clarity and Concentration:

Ingredients: 3 drops of mint, 3 drops of rosemary, 3 drops of lemon, 2 drops of cypress

Properties and Benefits: This blend is stimulating and refreshing, helping to improve concentration and mental clarity. Mint and rosemary are known to increase mental energy, while lemon helps focus the mind and reduce fatigue. Cypress, in turn, offers stability and structure, creating an environment conducive to work and study.

Practical Uses: This blend can be used in a diffuser in the workspace or applied diluted to the temples and wrists for study times or tasks that require focus.

Breathing and Focusing Exercises with Specific Oils

Conscious breathing, combined with essential oils, is an effective tool for boosting emotional and mental well-being. Inhaling certain oils while practicing deep breathing not only helps the active compounds reach the brain quickly, but also improves concentration and facilitates emotional connection. Below are several breathing exercises that enhance the effects of essential oils.

Deep Relaxation Breathing with Lavender and Incense:

Instructions: Place one drop each of lavender and frankincense in the palms of your hands, rub together to warm the oil, then place your hands near your face. Close your eyes, inhale deeply for a count of five, hold for another five seconds, then exhale slowly. Repeat this cycle at least five times, focusing on the calming sensation that each breath brings.

Benefits: This exercise helps reduce emotional and physical tension, promoting deep calm. It is ideal to perform before going to sleep or after a tiring day.

Energizing Breath with Mint and Lemon:

Instructions: Apply one drop of peppermint and lemon to a tissue. Hold the tissue close to your nose and inhale rapidly in three-second intervals for one minute. Allow yourself to feel the renewed energy that the fresh, citrusy aromas bring to your mind and body.

Benefits: This exercise is great for overcoming mental or physical fatigue. Peppermint stimulates alertness and mint helps improve focus, which is perfect for times when you need an energy boost.

Focus and Clarity Breathwork with Rosemary and Cypress:

Instructions: Place one drop each of rosemary and cypress in a diffuser or personal inhaler. Take long, slow breaths, inhaling for four seconds, holding for two, and exhaling for six seconds. As you inhale, visualize how each breath clears your mind and helps you focus.

Benefits: This exercise is excellent for improving mental clarity and reducing distraction. It can be done at the beginning of the day or before facing tasks that require high concentration.

Introspective Questions to Connect with Emotions Through Aromatherapy

Aromatherapy, combined with introspection, becomes a powerful practice of emotional healing and self-knowledge. The following introspective questions, accompanied by the application of essential oils, help the reader to deepen their emotional state and better understand their inner needs and desires. These questions can be used at the beginning or end of an aromatherapy session, while inhaling a specific aroma that encourages introspection.

Questions to Calm the Mind and Reduce Anxiety:

With Lavender or Frankincense: As you inhale a calming aroma, ask yourself, "What thoughts are making me anxious right now? Is there anything I can let go of or simplify in my life?"

With Ylang-Ylang: As you smell this balancing aroma, reflect: "What aspects of my life are causing me unnecessary stress? What can I do to restore peace and balance?"

Questions to Improve Mood and Self-Esteem:

With Bergamot or Rose: As you inhale an uplifting blend, ask yourself, "What do I need to feel happy and complete? Am I being compassionate to myself in my moments of weakness?"

With Geranium or Sweet Orange: These aromas help open the heart and encourage a positive outlook. Ask: "What aspects of my life bring me joy and gratitude? How can I nurture these aspects to enhance my well-being?"

Questions for Mental Clarity and Decision Making:

With Rosemary or Lemon: With these stimulating aromas, reflect: "What is my goal right now? What can I do to move toward that goal without distraction?"

With Mint and Cypress: As you breathe deeply into these aromas, ask yourself, "What thoughts or patterns do I need to let go of to improve my focus? What can I do today to live with clarity and purpose?"

How to Integrate the Use of Essential Oils into Your Daily Mental Wellness Routine

Aromatherapy becomes a more effective and meaningful practice when it is integrated into the daily routine. This allows the body and mind to associate certain aromas with specific moods, facilitating emotional adaptation throughout the day.

Below are suggestions for incorporating essential oils into your daily life and consistently reap their benefits:

Beginning and End of Day Rituals:

Morning: Use a blend of mint and lemon in a diffuser to start your day with energy and clarity. This practice helps you get into a state of alertness and focus right from the start of the day.

At Night: Place a blend of lavender and incense in a diffuser an hour before bed to create a calm and serene environment. This helps the transition to sleep and reduces the stress accumulated during the day.

Application Points for a Constant Effect:

Essential oils can be applied diluted to pulse points such as the wrists, neck, or behind the ears. This application allows the scent to linger and provide constant emotional support throughout the day.

Example: Applying a mixture of rose and geranium on the wrists is ideal for moments of emotional tension, as its aroma helps to open the heart and encourage a positive attitude.

Using Essential Oils in the Workspace:

Diffusing a blend of rosemary and cypress in your workspace helps maintain focus and concentration. If your work requires creativity, oils like frankincense and bergamot can also be used to inspire new ideas and reduce mental fatigue.

Example of Use: In projects or tasks that require creativity and clarity, the aromas of mint and lemon can promote open-mindedness and clear thinking, allowing the user to access their full potential.

PART III

AROMATHERAPY IN PHYSICAL HEALTH AND HOME

CHAPTER 5

AROMATHERAPY FOR PHYSICAL WELL-BEING

Essential oils not only influence the emotional state, but also have direct applications in physical well-being. These natural compounds have proven effective in relieving muscle discomfort, improving sleep quality, and promoting natural, chemical-free skin and hair care. This chapter explains how to harness the benefits of essential oils to improve physical health, from relieving pain and inflammation to improving rest and the vitality of skin and hair.

<u>Oils and Blends to Relieve Physical and Muscular Pain</u>

Aromatherapy is a valuable resource for relieving muscle and physical pain. Essential oils can help reduce inflammation, improve circulation and relieve muscle tension when applied topically or inhaled. Below are some of the most effective essential oils and some recommended blends for treating various types of pain.

Anti-inflammatory Oils:

Peppermint: The menthol present in peppermint essential oil provides a cooling sensation and helps reduce muscle pain and inflammation. It is especially useful for treating headaches and migraines if applied to the temples or back of the neck, diluted in a carrier oil.

Eucalyptus: This oil is known for its anti-inflammatory and analgesic properties, especially effective in relieving muscle and joint pain.

In addition, it's refreshing aroma helps clear the airways, making it an excellent choice for treating colds and associated aches and pains.

Rosemary: With circulation-stimulating properties, rosemary oil helps reduce muscle pain, tension and cramps. Applied in massage, it promotes muscle relaxation and is especially beneficial for lower back or shoulder pain.

Warming Blend for Muscle Tension:

Ingredients: 4 drops rosemary, 3 drops ginger, 2 drops mint, 1 drop black pepper

Use: Dilute in 10 ml of coconut or almond oil and apply to the affected area with a gentle massage. This mixture helps reduce tension and inflammation, providing a warm sensation that relaxes the muscles.

Refreshing Blend for Joint Pain:

Ingredients: 3 drops of mint, 3 drops of eucalyptus, 2 drops of lavender.

Use: Mix in 10 ml of aloe vera gel or a base oil and apply to painful joints. This combination has a cooling effect that reduces inflammation and improves comfort in the affected areas.

Aromatherapy for Rest and Restful Sleep

Sleep is one of the foundations of physical and mental health, and lack of rest can seriously affect overall well-being. Essential oils can be great allies to improve the quality of sleep, as they relax the nervous system and help reduce stress and anxiety. Here are some essential oils known for their relaxing properties and how to use them to achieve a deep rest.

Oils to Promote Sleep:

Lavender: This oil is one of the most well-known for its relaxing properties. Lavender reduces activity in the nervous system, helping to induce sleep and improve its quality. Inhaling lavender before bed has been shown to increase the amount of deep sleep.

Cedarwood: With a warm, earthy aroma, Cedarwood is ideal for creating a calming environment. This oil acts as a natural sedative, helping to reduce intrusive thoughts that can affect sleep.

Roman Chamomile: This oil is perfect for those who have difficulty relaxing before bed, as it helps calm the mind and relax the body.

Aromatherapy Rituals for Sleep:

Bedroom Diffuser: Place 5-7 drops of a blend of lavender, cedarwood, and Roman chamomile in an aromatherapy diffuser and turn it on an hour before bedtime. This allows the scent to disperse throughout the room, creating an environment conducive to rest.

Relaxing Pillow Spray:

Ingredients: 10 drops of lavender, 5 drops of cedar, 5 drops of bergamot, 100 ml of distilled water

Preparation and Use: Mix essential oils with distilled water in a spray bottle. Shake well before each use and spray on pillow and sheets to help relax before bed.

Skin and Hair Care with Essential Oils

Essential oils not only benefit the mind and body but can also be integrated into skin and hair care routines. Thanks to their antioxidant, antimicrobial and soothing properties, essential oils help improve the health and appearance of skin and hair naturally and effectively.

Skin Care Oils:

Rosehip: Rich in essential fatty acids and antioxidants, rosehip oil is ideal for skin regeneration, helping to reduce scars, blemishes and signs of aging.

Tea Tree: With antimicrobial and anti-inflammatory properties, tea tree is one of the most effective essential oils for treating acne and skin blemishes.

Geranium: This oil balances sebum production and improves the appearance of the skin, especially in combination or oily skin.

Moisturizing Skin Blend:

Ingredients: 3 drops of geranium, 2 drops of lavender, 2 drops of incense, 30 ml of jojoba oil

Use: Apply a small amount of this mixture to your face before going to bed. This formula deeply moisturizes the skin and helps improve its elasticity and luminosity.

Hair Care Oils:

Rosemary: This oil stimulates hair growth and strengthens hair, reducing hair loss. It is especially beneficial for people with fine or weakened hair.

Ylang-Ylang: Helps balance sebum production on the scalp and adds shine to the hair. It is ideal for those with dry or brittle hair.

Mint: Provides a refreshing sensation that stimulates circulation in the scalp, promoting healthy hair growth.

Hair Tonic for Hair Growth and Health:

Ingredients: 5 drops of rosemary, 3 drops of mint, 2 drops of ylang-ylang, 30 ml of distilled water

Use: Apply the tonic to the scalp and massage gently. It does not need rinsing and can be used two to three times a week to strengthen the hair and stimulate its growth.

CHAPTER 6

AROMATHERAPY IN THE HOME ENVIRONMENT

A harmonious and healthy home can be achieved through aromatherapy. Essential oils are powerful tools to purify the environment, create an energizing space, and offer natural, eco-friendly cleaning options. In this chapter, we will learn how to transform the home into a sanctuary of wellness using essential oils.

Creating a Harmonious Home Using Essential Oils

The environment in which we live directly influences our emotional and mental state. Aromatherapy allows us to create an environment that promotes well-being, whether through relaxing, revitalizing or balancing aromas. By choosing specific oils, it is possible to achieve an environment in harmony with our needs.

Oils for a Relaxing Environment:

Lavender: Calms the mind and reduces tension in the environment. It is ideal for relaxation or meditation areas.

Incense: Helps create a serene and spiritual atmosphere, ideal for moments of introspection and relaxation.

Oils for an Energizing Environment:

Lemon: Refreshes and revitalizes the space, providing a feeling of cleanliness and mental clarity.

Mint: Stimulates and refreshes the environment, ideal for study or work areas where concentration is required.

Environmental Diffuser:

Place a few drops of essential oil in an air diffuser to distribute the aromas throughout your home. This creates an atmosphere adapted to the activity you wish to carry out in each space.

Recipes for Environmental Purification and Space Energization

Essential oils can also be used to purify the air and energize the home. Here are some recipes to create a clean and lively environment:

Air Purifying Spray:

Ingredients: 10 drops of tea tree, 5 drops of eucalyptus, 5 drops of lemon, 100 ml of distilled water

Preparation and Use: Mix essential oils with water in a spray bottle. Shake well before each use and spray into the room to freshen the air and eliminate unwanted odors.

Energizing Home Blend:

Ingredients: 5 drops of orange, 5 drops of mint, 3 drops of rosemary

Use: Place the mixture in a diffuser and distribute in areas where a revitalizing atmosphere is desired, such as the living room or kitchen.

Oils for Natural and Ecological Cleaning at Home

Essential oils are an effective and eco-friendly alternative for home cleaning. Their antibacterial, antifungal and antiviral properties make them natural tools for disinfecting and cleaning without the use of harsh chemicals.

Multipurpose Cleaning:

Ingredients: 10 drops of tea tree, 5 drops of lemon, 100 ml of white vinegar, 200 ml of distilled water

Preparation and Use: Mix all ingredients in a spray bottle. This multi-purpose cleaner is ideal for disinfecting kitchen and bathroom surfaces naturally.

Floor Cleaning:

Ingredients: 10 drops of lavender, 10 drops of eucalyptus, 250 ml of distilled water

Preparation and Use: Mix essential oils with water in a bucket and use to clean floors. This solution leaves a fresh scent throughout the home and helps eliminate bacteria from the floor.

PART IV

SPIRITUAL AND ENERGETIC AROMATHERAPY

CHAPTER 7

ENERGY BALANCE AND AROMATHERAPY

Energy balancing is an important practice in many spiritual traditions, and aromatherapy fits perfectly into this process. Because of their vibrational properties, essential oils can be used to activate, balance and harmonize the chakras. In this chapter, we will delve into the symbolism and energy of each chakra and how certain oils can positively influence them to promote complete and lasting alignment.

Introduction to Energy and Chakras in Aromatherapy

Chakras represent energy points that, according to spiritual philosophies, affect our physical, emotional and spiritual health. Aromatherapy becomes a bridge to the balance of these energy centers, taking advantage of the natural vibration of essential oils. Each essential oil emits a frequency that resonates with the energy of a specific chakra, and when inhaled or applied to the body, this energy is absorbed, helping to balance and harmonize the associated chakra .

Root (Muladhara):

Energy and Symbolism : This chakra is linked to stability, security and our basic needs. It is related to red and represents the connection with the earth and the sense of belonging.

Oils and Rituals: Cedarwood and vetiver, with their earthy aromas, facilitate a feeling of grounding and connection to the ground. Visualizing a red light flowing from the base of the spine to the ground, while inhaling cedar, enhances this connection and reduces fear and insecurity.

Sacral (Svadhisthana):

Energy and Symbolism: This chakra is the center of creativity and emotions. Associated with orange, it is related to emotional expression and enjoyment of life.

Emotional Expression Oils and Practices: Sandalwood and ylang-ylang oils help open the energetic flow of this chakra , allowing for healthy emotional expression. A free-flowing ritual can be performed by applying ylang-ylang to the abdomen, which helps release repressed emotions and promotes creativity.

Solar Plexus (Manipura):

Energy and Symbolism: This yellow chakra represents self-confidence, personal power and will. A balanced solar plexus helps you make firm decisions and act with determination.

Strengthening Oils and Practices: Ginger and rosemary oils are ideal for stimulating personal power and vital energy. Applying ginger to the solar plexus and taking deep breaths while visualizing a radiant sun increases confidence and self-control.

Heart (Anahata):

Energy and Symbolism: The heart chakra is related to love, compassion and empathy. Its green color symbolizes growth and openness towards others.

Oils for Love and Empathy: Rose essential oil is particularly powerful for opening this chakra and stimulating unconditional love. Placing a few drops of rose on your chest and inhaling deeply while visualizing a halo of green light around your heart facilitates forgiveness and emotional connection.

Throat (Vishuddha):

Energy and Symbolism: This light blue chakra is associated with expression, communication, and authenticity. It represents our ability to speak the truth and listen to others.

Communication Oils and Exercises: Peppermint and eucalyptus oils open the throat chakra, helping to express thoughts and emotions clearly. Applying peppermint to the throat and reciting affirmations of authenticity out loud improves communication skills and self-confidence.

Third Eye (Ajna):

Energy and Symbolism : This chakra , indigo in color, is linked to intuition, perception and inner wisdom. A balanced third eye allows one to see beyond appearances and understand the truth.

Oils for Clarity and Intuition: Lavender and frankincense are ideal for opening the third eye and developing intuition. Placing a few drops of lavender between the eyebrows while meditating and visualizing an eye of light helps to deepen perception and intuition.

Crown (Sahasrara):

Energy and Symbolism: This violet chakra represents spiritual connection and cosmic consciousness. Its activation promotes deep understanding and integration with the whole.

Oils for Spiritual Expansion: Frankincense and myrrh open the crown chakra, facilitating a deeper connection with the spiritual plane. Applying these oils to the crown of the head while performing a meditation to connect with the cosmic light helps to expand consciousness.

CHAPTER 8

OILS FOR MEDITATION AND SPIRITUAL PRACTICE

Meditation and other spiritual practices are enhanced by the use of essential oils that help create a sacred environment, increase mental clarity and promote a deeper connection to one's inner essence. Essential oils can act as guides for introspection and spiritual growth, and their intentional use brings peace, clarity and a sense of purpose.

Guide to Oils for Introspection and Self-Knowledge

For self-knowledge work, certain essential oils help create an atmosphere of calm and inner silence that facilitates the observation of thoughts and emotions from a place of acceptance. Below are the ideal oils for this practice and their applications in specific exercises.

Incense for Deep Spiritual Connection:

Uses and Properties: This oil, known as the "king of essential oils", helps a person reconnect with their inner spirit. Its aroma induces calm and clarity, promoting a calm and receptive mind.

Deep Reflection Exercise: Place incense in a diffuser or on a handkerchief and inhale while practicing long, conscious breathing. Visualize a sacred space within and let any thoughts or emotions arise without judgment.

Sandalwood for Peace and Stability:

Uses and Properties: Sandalwood is great for focusing the mind and providing emotional stability during introspection. It is known to help people find answers in silence.

Self-Acceptance Exercise: Apply a few drops of sandalwood to your chest or wrists before an introspective practice. Sit quietly and focus on your breathing, repeating an affirmation such as "I fully accept myself as I am."

Myrrh for Inner Wisdom:

Uses and Properties: Myrrh is an ancient oil that provides wisdom and understanding. Its dense and mystical aroma facilitates the encounter with one's own thoughts and emotions.

Visualization Exercise: Place myrrh in a diffuser and close your eyes, imagining a dark, quiet space where only your own consciousness exists. Allow any thoughts to develop and observe them with compassion and detachment.

Blends for Focus in Meditation and Mindfulness Practices

Essential oil blends are especially effective for meditation and mindfulness, as they amplify the individual benefits of each oil. The following formulas help to deepen meditation and keep your attention in the present.

Inner Peace Blend:

Ingredients: 4 drops of incense, 3 drops of lavender, 2 drops of sandalwood

Use: Place this blend in a diffuser at the beginning of your meditation. This combination helps create an atmosphere of deep peace, promoting mental serenity and emotional clarity.

Mindfulness Focus Blend:

Ingredients: 3 drops of rosemary, 3 drops of mint, 2 drops of eucalyptus

Use: Ideal for mindfulness practices, this blend helps keep your focus on the present. It can be applied to the wrists or inhaled before practice.

Exercises to Enhance Spiritual Connection Through Aroma

Spiritual exercises are enhanced when aromatherapy is incorporated, as the aroma acts as a portal to deepen the experience. The following exercises are designed to leverage essential oils for spiritual connection and inner growth.

Consciousness Expansion Meditation with Lotus and Incense:

Instructions: Place lotus and incense in a diffuser, sit comfortably and close your eyes. Visualize a light expanding from the heart to the entire being, allowing the aroma to accompany this expansion process. This helps to feel a deep connection with one's own essence and with the entire universe.

Spiritual Visualization Exercise with Cedar:

Instructions: Apply a drop of cedarwood to your palms, rub them together, and place your hands in front of your face, inhaling deeply. Close your eyes and visualize an ancient, sacred forest. The cedarwood aroma will help transport your mind to that sacred space and strengthen your connection to nature.

Ritual of Connection with the Inner Being using Rose and Myrrh:

Instructions: Apply a mixture of rose and myrrh to your chest and neck. Sit in a quiet place and breathe deeply, visualizing an encounter with your inner self. This ritual helps foster self-love and deep understanding, creating a space of peace and reconciliation with yourself.

PART V

SAFETY, ETHICS AND PRACTICES IN MODERN AROMATHERAPY

CHAPTER 9

THE SAFE USE OF ESSENTIAL OILS

Safety in the use of essential oils is essential to ensure a positive and beneficial aromatherapy experience. Although essential oils offer multiple benefits, their high concentration makes them powerful substances that require conscious and careful application. In this chapter, we will address precautions and recommendations for safe use, explore potential interactions with other treatments and medications, and discuss specific protocols for using oils around children, pets, and sensitive environments.

Precautions and Recommendations for Safe Application

Dilution and Dosage:

Importance of Dilution: Essential oils are extremely concentrated, so they must be diluted in a carrier oil before topical application. Proper dilution varies by oil and purpose, but a 1% to 5% dilution is generally recommended, depending on skin sensitivity and the area of the body to be applied.

Dosage in Diffusers: For use in diffusers, 5 to 10 drops per 100 ml of water is suggested, depending on the desired intensity and ventilation of the room. Excessive oil may irritate the respiratory tract or cause headaches.

Safe Topical Application:

Patch Test: Before applying a new essential oil to your skin, it is advisable to do a patch test. Place a small, diluted amount on your forearm and wait 24 hours to observe any possible reactions.

Avoid Sensitive Areas: Never apply essential oils directly to sensitive areas, such as eyes, mucous membranes, or genitals. Certain oils, such as citrus oils, can cause photosensitivity if applied to the skin before sun exposure.

Oils Ingestion:

Extreme Caution: Ingestion of essential oils should only be done under the supervision of a trained professional, as some oils can be toxic when ingested. In many cases, topical or diffused use is sufficient to obtain the desired benefits without risk of toxicity.

Interactions with Other Treatments and Medications

Possible Interactions:

Oils with Anticoagulant Effect: Some essential oils, such as clove and cinnamon, have anticoagulant properties and may interact with medications that alter coagulation, such as warfarin. This may increase the risk of bleeding in some people.

Sedative Oils: Lavender and chamomile, known for their relaxing effects, can enhance the effect of sedative medications, so they should be used with caution in people who are already taking tranquilizers or sedatives.

Consult with Health Professionals:

Medical Supervision: Individuals who are undergoing medication treatment, especially those with chronic illnesses or who take medications on an ongoing basis, should consult their physician or an aromatherapy professional before integrating essential oils into their routine.

Your healthcare provider can evaluate any potential interactions and adjust doses as needed.

Safety Protocols for Use Around Children, Pets and Sensitive Environments

Safe Use in Children:

Age-appropriate dilutions: Children's skin is more sensitive than that of adults, so the dilution should be even lower. For babies up to 6 months, it is recommended to avoid applying essential oils. For children from 6 months to 2 years, the dilution should be 0.25%-0.5%, and for children from 2 to 6 years, 1%.

Suitable Oils: Not all oils are safe for children; oils such as eucalyptus and rosemary, which contain cineole , can cause respiratory problems in children. Milder oils, such as lavender and chamomile, are safer options.

Safe Use in Pets:

Animal Sensitivity: Pets, especially cats, are extremely sensitive to essential oils, as their liver does not metabolize the compounds in the same way as a human's. Avoid oils such as tea tree, which is toxic to cats and dogs.

Diffusers in Shared Spaces: If using oils in diffusers in spaces where pets are present, it is important to ensure that the space is well ventilated and that pets have the option to leave the room if they wish.

Sensitive Environments and Vulnerable People:

People with Allergies and Sensitivities: Some people may be more sensitive to certain oils, so it is essential to do an initial test with a small amount of oil in the diffuser and observe possible reactions.

Elderly and Pregnant Women: Pregnant women and older adults should avoid certain oils, such as rosemary and sage, as they may affect the hormonal system or induce contractions. Gentle, low-dose oils are recommended for use under professional supervision.

CHAPTER 10

ETHICAL AND SUSTAINABLE AROMATHERAPY

The growing interest in aromatherapy has led to an expansion of essential oil production, but this has also put significant pressure on natural resources. In this context, ethical and sustainable practice becomes a responsibility for those who choose to include essential oils in their lives. In this chapter we will discuss how to choose responsibly sourced oils, support ethical and sustainable practices, and reduce the environmental impact of aromatherapy.

<u>Choosing Oils from Responsible Sources</u>

Transparency and Traceability:

Importance of Traceability: It is essential to know the origin of the essential oil you purchase. Choosing suppliers who share detailed information about the origin of their oils guarantees higher quality and ensures that ethical practices are followed in production.

Certifications: Look for essential oils that have fair trade, organic, and sustainability certifications. These certifications ensure that production respects both workers and the environment, ensuring a positive impact.

Sustainable Cultivation and Harvesting Practices:

Ethical and Regenerative Harvesting: Some essential oils require large amounts of plant material to produce, such as sandalwood and rose. To protect the environment, it is important to choose brands that adopt sustainable harvesting practices, reforest the plants used, and allow for their regeneration.

Collaboration with Local Communities: Responsible companies often collaborate with local communities, promoting the local economy and respecting traditional knowledge about the cultivation and use of aromatic plants.

How to Support Ethical and Sustainable Practices in Aromatherapy

Consumer Education and Awareness:

Product Knowledge: Consumer education is essential to promote ethical practices. Understanding how oils are produced, and the impact of each crop allows for more informed and conscious decisions.

Support Ethical Suppliers: Choosing brands that are committed to ethical and sustainable practices helps promote a more conscious and respectful marketplace. Researching and reading reviews about companies before purchasing can make a huge difference.

Rational Use of Oils:

Use in Moderately and Consciously: Essential oils are extremely concentrated and potent, so it is not necessary to use large quantities to obtain benefits. Using only the necessary amount reduces demand and decreases the pressure on natural resources.

Recycling Packaging: Opting for reusable or recyclable packaging is another way to reduce your environmental impact. Some brands offer recycling programs for their packaging, which helps minimize waste.

Environmental Impact and How to Reduce It

Reducing the Ecological Footprint:

Responsible Production: The production of essential oils can be resource intensive. For example, producing one liter of rose essential oil requires thousands of rose petals. Supporting brands that use responsible cultivation methods helps reduce pressure on ecosystems.

Moderate Use of Resources: Limiting the use of essential oils and opting for less intensive methods, such as using diffusers instead of baths, can reduce the impact on the environment.

Promotion of Biodiversity:

Sustainable Harvesting and Support for Reforestation: Some brands partner with reforestation organizations to replenish harvested plants. These initiatives promote biodiversity and help conserve species at risk of overexploitation.

Diversification of Aromatic Plants: Instead of focusing solely on popular oils, such as lavender or eucalyptus, consumers can explore other less common oils that offer similar benefits. This reduces the pressure on specific species and encourages biodiversity.

CONCLUSION

Aromatherapy is much more than wellness practice; it is a gateway to a deeper connection with oneself, the environment, and nature. Throughout this book, we have explored the richness of essential oils from multiple perspectives: their physical and emotional impact, their ability to balance energy and enhance the home environment, and their contribution to spirituality and awareness. This conclusion serves as an invitation to integrate aromatherapy in a conscious and respectful way, honoring its power and origin.

Reflection on the Conscious and Respectful Use of Aromatherapy

The essence of aromatherapy is based on the ability of scents to transform our inner state and connect us with nature. However, it is important to remember that each bottle of essential oil represents a significant effort by nature and by those who grow, harvest and distill the plants. By using essential oils consciously and moderately, we commit to respecting these precious resources and valuing their provenance and the energy of the plants that originate them.

Valuation of Natural Resources:

Each essential oil is the result of a careful and respectful extraction process, which often involves using large amounts of raw material. This knowledge leads us to use oils thoughtfully and to choose brands that practice sustainable methods. Thus, by using these oils, we not only gain personal benefits, but we also contribute to practices that respect and protect the planet.

Caution and Moderation in Use:

Conscious aromatherapy involves not only choosing good quality oils, but also using them in moderation. The high concentration of essential oils means that a small amount is sufficient to achieve significant effects. Practicing moderation not only extends the shelf life of each bottle, but also decreases production requirements and reduces our impact on the environment.

Commitment to Ethical Practices:

The growing demand for essential oils poses challenges for the environment and for the communities that produce them. By choosing ethical suppliers committed to sustainability, we support a supply chain that benefits all parties involved. This choice reflects a commitment to holistic well-being that takes into account the impact of our actions beyond our own benefit.

Invitation to a Comprehensive Wellness Practice

Aromatherapy has the potential to enrich the lives of those who practice it, not only as a resource for physical and emotional health, but also as a path to holistic wellness. The invitation is to explore aromatherapy as a tool for self-knowledge, healing and connection, integrating its benefits into all aspects of daily life.

Emotional and Spiritual Wellbeing:

Essential oils can be a powerful tool for cultivating calm, reducing stress and fostering connection with the inner self. Through practices such as meditation, mindfulness and introspection, it is possible to deepen self-knowledge and understanding of our emotions. The invitation is to discover how oils can support personal growth and spiritual evolution, creating a space of peace and balance in daily life.

Connection with the Environment:

Aromatherapy allows us to create a harmonious atmosphere at home and at work, improving the quality of the space we inhabit. By using oils to purify the environment, relax the mind or revitalize the body, we contribute to creating an atmosphere that reflects the well-being we desire for ourselves and those around us. The invitation is to consider each space as a sanctuary and to incorporate the aromas that best meet the needs of each moment.

Holistic and Balanced Practice:

Aromatherapy, used consciously, is not an isolated practice, but an integral part of a holistic approach to wellness. In combination with healthy eating, physical exercise, adequate rest and emotional care practices, essential oils become a resource that complements and supports the balance of body, mind and spirit. The final invitation is to view aromatherapy not only as a wellness practice, but as a philosophy of life that reminds us of the importance of caring for ourselves and the natural world around us.

Additional Resources for Those Who Wish to Delve Deeper into the Science and Spirituality of Aromas

For those who wish to continue their exploration of aromatherapy, there are numerous resources and tools that allow you to delve deeper into both the science of essential oils and their spiritual dimension. The following resources offer a starting point to expand your knowledge and continue to discover the potential of this practice.

Books and Scientific Publications:

The Complete Guide to Aromatherapy by Salvatore Battaglia: This book is one of the most comprehensive texts on aromatherapy, offering a detailed look at both the scientific and spiritual aspects of essential oils.

Essential Oil Safety by Robert Tisserand and Rodney Young: An essential guide to the safe use of oils, based on scientific research and studies on toxicity, interactions, and precautions.

The Healing Intelligence of Essential Oils by Kurt Schnaubelt: A more spiritual and holistic approach, exploring how essential oils can support personal growth and healing.

Aromatherapy Training and Certification:

There are aromatherapy training programs, both in-person and online, that provide in-depth, accredited knowledge of the use of essential oils. Some of the world-renowned organizations are *Aromahead Institute,* the *National Association for Holistic Aromatherapy (NAHA)* and the *Pacific Institute of Aromatherapy.* These programs are an excellent option for those who wish to practice aromatherapy professionally or as a personal development discipline.

Online Communities and Support Groups:

Online communities dedicated to aromatherapy are spaces where aromatherapy enthusiasts can share experiences, knowledge and advice. Pages like *Aromatherapy United* and social media groups allow you to connect with people around the world who share a passion for aromatherapy and offer a place to ask questions and learn from the experiences of others.

Scientific Research Resources and New Trends:

As the science of aromatherapy continues to evolve, there are more and more studies and publications on the therapeutic benefits of essential oils. Sites such as *PubMed* and *ResearchGate* publish recent research exploring the properties of oils and their medical and psychological applications. These resources allow readers to stay up to date and learn about advancements in the field of aromatherapy.

<u>Final Words</u>

Aromatherapy, in essence, is a practice of connection and respect. It connects us to ourselves, to our emotions and to the natural world, of which essential oils are an expression. By integrating scents into our daily lives, we also deepen our respect for nature and recognize the impact our choices have on it.

As we say goodbye, we invite you to continue exploring this path of self-knowledge and healing, always remembering that every scent, every oil and every inhalation is an opportunity to live with greater balance and harmony. May this book guide you on your journey and may each drop of essential oil you use be an invitation to live with awareness and gratitude.

APPENDICES

APPENDIX A

GLOSSARY OF TERMS IN AROMATHERAPY

The language of aromatherapy includes specific terms that may be new to beginners or have meanings in this field. Below you will find a glossary that clarifies some of the key concepts, facilitating a better understanding of aromatherapy terminology.

Carrier Oil: A vegetable oil used to dilute essential oils before topical application. Common examples include almond oil, jojoba oil, and fractionated coconut oil.

Antimicrobial: Property of an essential oil that helps fight or inhibit the growth of microorganisms such as bacteria, fungi and viruses.

Cineole: Natural compound found in some oils, such as eucalyptus, known for its anti-inflammatory and decongestant properties.

Diffusion: Method of dispersing essential oils into the air using a diffuser, humidifier or oil burner for inhalation and aromatherapy.

Dilution: The process of combining essential oils with carrier oils to reduce their concentration and make them safe for topical application.

Photosensitivity: Skin reaction to sun exposure, which is intensified by some essential oils (such as citrus oils), which can cause irritation or spots on the skin.

Aromatic Note: Classification of essential oils according to the duration and intensity of their aroma, which can be high, medium or low (also known as top, heart and base notes).

Chemotype: Chemical variation within a plant species that results in differences in its properties. Some oils, such as rosemary, have multiple chemotypes with different therapeutic applications.

Synergy: Intensified effect obtained by combining two or more essential oils, resulting in benefits greater than those each oil would have separately.

Olfactory pathway: Route through which aromas, when inhaled, reach the brain and generate a physiological or emotional response.

APPENDIX B

TABLE OF ESSENTIAL OILS AND THEIR PROPERTIES

1. Calming and Relaxing Oils

Lavender:

Properties: Calming, anti-inflammatory, sedative.

Main Uses: Anxiety reduction, help with insomnia, relief of skin irritation.

Ylang-Ylang:

Properties: Relaxing, harmonizing, aphrodisiac.

Main Uses: Emotional balance, relaxation, hair care.

Roman Chamomile:

Properties: Soothing, anti-inflammatory.

Main Uses: Anxiety reduction, menstrual discomfort relief, sensitive skin care.

2. Energizing and Stimulating Oils

Mint:

Properties: Refreshing, stimulating, decongestant.

Main Uses: Relief of fatigue, treatment of headaches, nasal decongestion.

Lemon:

Properties: Energizing, antimicrobial, astringent.

Main Uses: Energy and mental clarity, home cleaning, environmental purification.

Rosemary:

Properties: Stimulating, clarifying, antiseptic.

Main Uses: Improved concentration, hair growth, muscle pain relief.

3. Oils for Purification and Cleansing

Tea Tree:

Properties: Antibacterial, antifungal, antiviral.

Main Uses: Treatment of acne, skin infections, surface cleansing.

Eucalyptus:

Properties: Decongestant, antimicrobial.

Main Uses: Relief of colds, sinusitis, environmental purification.

Lemon (also in the energizer category):

Main Uses: Home cleaning, surface purification, natural air freshener.

4. Oils for Meditation and Spirituality

Incense:

Properties: Spiritual, relaxing, anti-inflammatory.

Main Uses: Meditation, skin care, scar reduction.

Sandalwood:

Properties: Stabilizing, calming.

Main Uses: Meditation, emotional balance, spiritual strengthening.

Myrrh:

Properties: Antiseptic, spiritual, calming.

Primary Uses: Meditation, spiritual connection, emotional protection.

5. Balancing Oils for Emotional Well-Being

Geranium:

Properties: Balancing, antiseptic, anti-inflammatory.

Main Uses: Stress reduction, hormonal balance, skin care.

Pink:

Properties: Soothing, moisturizing, revitalizing

Main Uses: Anxiety reduction, dry skin treatment, emotional balance.

Cedar:

Properties: Rooting , antiseptic, calming.

Main Uses: Anxiety, energy balance, hair care.

APPENDIX C

RESOURCES AND RECOMMENDED READINGS FOR FURTHER STUDY

For those who wish to expand their knowledge of aromatherapy, both scientific and spiritual aspects, here is a list of books, courses, and online sources that offer more advanced training.

Recommended Books:

The Complete Book of Essential Oils and Aromatherapy by Valerie Ann Worwood: A comprehensive handbook on the uses of essential oils in various aspects of life, from health to emotional well-being.

Essential Oil Safety: A Guide for Health Care Professionals by Robert Tisserand and Rodney Young: An indispensable resource for learning about the safe use of oils, based on detailed scientific research.

The Art of Aromatherapy by Robert Tisserand: An exploration of the traditional and spiritual uses of essential oils, from a historical and holistic perspective.

Aromatherapy Organizations and Certifications:

National Association for Holistic Aromatherapy (NAHA) : One of the most recognized organizations for aromatherapy education . Offers courses and certifications, as well as an extensive library of online resources.

Aromahead Institute: Aromatherapy training institute offering online courses with certification, ideal for both beginners and professionals.

Journals and Scientific Publications:

Journal of Essential Oil Research: Academic publication that presents studies and advances in the field of essential oils, including research on their therapeutic and chemical applications.

PubMed: Scientific research database where you can find clinical studies and reviews on the effects and safety of essential oils.

Online Resources:

Aromatherapy United: Online community offering articles, guides, and discussion forums on ethical and sustainable practices in aromatherapy.

ResearchGate and Google Scholar: Platforms where you can access recent scientific studies on the therapeutic effects of essential oils and their chemical properties.

ACKNOWLEDGEMENTS

To all those who have contributed to making this work possible, from the professionals who shared their knowledge to those who provided support and encouragement at every stage of the process.

Thank you for your time, dedication and enthusiasm. Your contribution was invaluable in enriching these pages and bringing the wisdom of aromatherapy to more people. This project is also a reflection of your generosity and commitment.